MOTHER OF THE WORLD

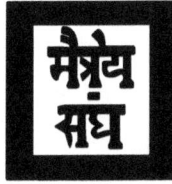

MOTHER OF
THE WORLD

FROM AGNI YOGA TEACHINGS

AGNI YOGA SOCIETY

2019

Agni Yoga Society
319 West 107th Street
New York NY 10025
www.agniyoga.org

ISBN: 978-0-933574-17-5

Dedicated to all who look for the Coming of the Great Teacher foretold by Gautama Buddha—The Lord Maitreya—Christ, Buddha, spiritual Guide, Leader of the New Race—Who has given to humanity a new revelation of the World Mother.

MOTHER OF THE WORLD

Selections from the books of the
Agni Yoga Teachings for the New Era

- *Leaves of Morya's Garden I, The Call,* 1924
- *Leaves of Morya's Garden II, Illumination,* 1925
- *New Era Community,* 1926
- *Agni Yoga,* 1929
- *Infinity I,* 1930
- *Hierarchy,* 1931
- *Heart,* 1932
- *Fiery World I,* 1933
- *Fiery World II,* 1934
- *Fiery World III,* 1935
- *Aum,* 1936
- *Letters of Helena Roerich,* 1929-1938, Volume I

FOREWORD (1956)

IN the Hermetic Writings of old are found references to "the Woman clothed with the Sun." Is this a symbol or a sublime Reality of the Higher World?

Ancient religions, inspired by Messengers of the Planetary Hierarchy, accorded great reverence to the Feminine Principle in Creation, the Mother aspect of Deity.

The highest manifestation of this Feminine Principle has been called by many names, among them, Mother of the Universe, World Mother, Isis, Ishtar, and Sophia. To the Gnostic Christians She was known as the Holy Spirit, one of the Divine Triad; but ecclesiastical Christianity has regarded the Holy Trinity as entirely masculine, thus depriving its adherents of a sublime and ennobling Concept.

In the following pages will be found selections from the Teachings of Living Ethics—given by the Lord Maitreya—which illumine the Image of this Majestic Being, the Matriarch and Initiator of the Planetary Hierarchy, the spiritual Mother of all the Christs and Buddhas of human history—the spiritual Mother also of every child of Earth whose heart is attuned to Her's.

MOTHER OF THE WORLD

Leaves of Morya's Garden Vol. I, The Call

357. They are rending the Raiment of the Lord.
They scoff at its tatters.
But the daughter of the world and the Mother of
the Universe will join the pieces of this Raiment.
And thou wilt come ready to receive thy vestment.
For, wherefore the power and wherefore the sacrifice,
if there be no joy?
And where is compassion,
And where is devotion,
And where is the love of creation,
If thy shoulders are not bedecked with the
Raiment of the Mother of the World?

Leaves of Morya's Garden Vol. Il, Illumination

150. The Mother of the World appears as a symbol of the Feminine Origin in the New Epoch, and the Masculine Origin voluntary returns the treasure of the World to the Feminine Origin.

153. The Star of the Morning is the sign of the Great Epoch which will flash as the first ray from the Teaching of Christ. For who is to extol the Mother of the World if not Christ, Who was so demeaned by the world?

220. I have already told you that the Mother of the World conceals Her Name. I have already shown you how the Mother of the World veils Her Face. I have already made mention about the Mother of Buddha and Christ.

Indeed it is time to point out that the one Mother of both Lords is not a symbol but a great manifestation of the Feminine Origin, in which is revealed the spiritual Mother of Christ and Buddha.

She it was Who taught and ordained Them for achievement.

From times immemorial the Mother of the World has sent forth to achievement. In the history of humanity, Her Hand traces an unbreakable thread.

On Sinai Her Voice rang out. She assumed the image of Kali. She was at the basis of the cults of Isis and Ishtar. After Atlantis, when a blow was inflicted upon the cult of the spirit, the Mother of the World began to weave a new thread, which will now begin to radiate. After Atlantis the Mother of the World veiled Her Face and forbade the pronouncement of Her Name until the hour of the constellations should strike. She has manifested Herself only partly; never has She manifested Herself on a planetary scale.

221. Now, more about the Mother of the World.

The Mother is Beauty; the world is self-sacrifice. Precisely by these two fundamentals are the Gates opened.

232. The spheres of the elements are of dazzling beauty, and besmirching them is like destroying a wonderful flower. I feel that the teaching of pure thoughts will penetrate into people's consciousness. The sower of thought gathers the harvest. Therefore, with the Mother of the World all-seeing cooperation is unavoidable. The

state of the substance of the space, pierced by the combinations of new rays, permits the beginning of the New Era. All Good should be gathered.

301. Let the things of everyday life vanish, but let the country of the future be embodied in thought. And what cleanses the spirit more thoroughly than thoughts about the welfare of others? And what tempers the armor of steadfastness better than the wish to lead others to Light? And what weaves a better smile than a desire to see the very last child laughing? I urge you to think thus about the future, to place daily a pearl into the necklace of the Mother of the World. And so, concisely and simply think how to adorn the Hearth of the World.

350. You have already heard about the saturation of rhythm of labor as a particular quality possessed but rarely by people. Its beneficial influence has a far deeper significance than it may appear to have. Yet the ancient mysteries used these two expressions: "to labor in the wave of Sublime Nature" and "to work with the heartbeat of the Mother of the World."

New Era Community

21. We are not lovers of the world of bodily survivals, the lower Subtle World—the Astral World— but, like everything else that exists, it cannot be avoided in spiritual development. The world of bodily survivals contains certain elements needed for the intercourse between the worlds. For example, the means of transportation are very little understood by the dwellers of the Subtle World. Although they have the possibility to strive upwards they are busy with the constructing of dark houses, in imitation of the earthly ones. But if

still during their lifetime they had broadened their consciousnesses, they would have been able to measure the hem of the garment of the Mother of the World.

72. The Community, as Fellowship, can unprecedentedly accelerate the evolution of the planet and give new possibilities of intercourse with the forces of matter. It must not be thought that community and the conquest of matter are found on different planes. One channel, one banner—Maitreya, Mother, Matter!

78. Mother and Teacher—these two concepts must be safeguarded in each book. The light of greatness is not to be extinguished.

216. In Our Hindu writings you have encountered the expression "play" applied to cosmic concepts. The play of the Great Mother of the World—is it not visible to the illumined consciousness? And the drama of blood—is it not changed in the light of radiant matter? Yet for the radiant play it is necessary to have a prepared hour.

224. Indeed, creativeness is diffused throughout all labor, and some sparks of great "Aum" direct the current of life. That manifestation of creative power forms the nodes of evolution, and through it is fastened the thread of the Mother of the World, fastened in a labor of eternal action.

Agni Yoga

20. Rejoice in the Great Play of the Mother of the World!

55. The old world rejected the Mother of the World, but the New World begins to perceive Her lustrous veil.

60. How great is the play of the Mother of the World! She beckons to Her children from far-distant fields:

"Hasten, children! I wish to teach you. I have keen eyes and alert ears ready for you. Sit ye down upon My garment. Let us learn to soar!"

64. Our Brothers may sometimes be seen by you with Their faces not clearly visible. If the face is somewhat misty, you may be assured that that Person is immersed in a lengthy experiment that requires a fixation of the gaze in one direction. If a woman's figure is seen with a veiled face, this manifestation relates to the Mother of the World.

72. Have you finally learned to rejoice at obstacles? Can We be assured that the seeming obstacle will tenfold multiply your resourcefulness? Can We term you conquering warriors? Can We send you the arrow of help, assured that you will catch it in flight? Can We pronounce the word of the New World in unison with you? Can We believe that for the sake of the beauty of creation you have burned your outworn garments? Can the Mother of the World entrust to your vigilance the texture of Light? Can the "Lion" hasten to your aid? Can the Light illumine your way? Victory knocks. And finally, do you understand how to apply to yourself the given Teaching? Can We trust you with the wearing of the given signs? Can We dispatch the ray of perfectment? Can We vouch for your vigilance? Can We construct a rampart from your understanding of self? Can We rejoice at the steadfastness of your path? Can the Mother of the World name you the just? Could the "Lion" become the guard at your dwelling? Can the Light bathe the new steps? Unbolt your portals!

82. Can one trust a blind helmsman? Can one think that the rags of antiquated thought may be utilized for

the New World? One must understand that the gift of the New World will be brought to the open gates. Verily, the New World wishes to bestow a beautiful garment. Approach, humanity, and receive the texture, fashioned by the labor of the Mother of the World!

142. Let us take the example of a structure. For the construction of the new house the old building is demolished. Each stone, each beam removed from the old nest, cries against the injustice of the act. But the dismemberment has taken place and new energy has flared up. Kali, the Destroyer, has become Mother, the Creator. Out of the fragments a new structure is built. New energy floods the space. With such simple examples one should remember the need of the regeneration of energy.

163. As sculptors, begin to touch the different surfaces of the raw matter. Thus, suddenly and continuously strike sparks of the Fire of Life from the surface of chaos. As the play of the Great Mother gathers power in the spiral curves of the energy of Fohat, thus fearlessly give people a complete, though unexpected, understanding of uniting all life in the realization of the Infinite.

306. The Breath of the Mother of the World, the Giants bearing the Burden, and the Redeemers who have accepted the chalice—these three images were born close to the one law. The cumulation of psychic energy of space creates explosions in parts of the planet. The organisms which attune to the Breath of the Great Mother, reverberate in response to the explosions of the bodies of space. Can such a tremor be regarded as an advantage? It is precisely as when, for the execution of a superb creation, one chooses perfectly attuned instruments. Of course, when such instruments are few the

pressure of the currents lies upon those few. Although it is needless to prove it, nevertheless it is better to accept the burden of the world than to be detached from the life of action.

315. The Mother of the World has ordained: "Winds, gather ye! Snows, gather ye! Birds, hold ye back! Beasts, stand ye back!

"No human foot shall set its traces on My Summit. The audacity of the dark ones shall not surmount! The light of the moon shall not endure! But the sun rays shall touch the Peak.

"Sun, guard My Summit, because where else shall I keep My Vigil? Never shall beast ascend, nor shall human power prevail!"

Herself, the Mother of all Being, shall keep Her Vigil with a fiery shield. What glows upon the Summit? Why have the whirlwinds assembled a resplendent crown?

She, the Great Mother, alone ascended the Summit. And none shall follow Her.

317. Upon the highest summit stands effulgent the Mother of the World. She came forth to smite the darkness. Why are the enemies fallen? And whither do they turn their eyes in desperation? She has cloaked Herself in a fiery mantle and encircled Herself in a fiery wall. She is our citadel and our striving.

326. Every structure has its outer walls and its invisible foundation. One cannot be without walls, but walls will not stand without foundation. There are two aspects of manifestation in everything: one is the walls, as a symbol of the Teacher, and the other is the foundation, as the manifestation of the Mother of the World. Which is more substantial? Ponder!

327. The walls and the pillars of foundation are equally necessary for the building. If the pillar of foundation is unseen from afar, then also the image of the Mother of the World remains invisible. The walls take on themselves the assaults of the gale. Our Name is given out to multitudes, but We accept the assaults of the hostile currents.

376. How do We regard success? Verily, the works are successful because their very trail is followed by both friends and foes. Trace the record of imitations and say to yourself, "all issues from our fire." The mistakes are drowned in the successive fires. One may boldly swim when the fires of the beacons are projected, when the dangers are manifesting the design of the Veil of the Mother of the World.

The Mother of the World does not fear the Great Play.

377. Let us count the days spent unworthily and be stricken with terror. Let us count the hours not given to the Teaching and bewail. Can one sell the hour of Teaching for a sack of gold? Can one be reconciled to the garment of ignorance after beholding a chiton of beauty adorned with the flowers of the Mother of the World? How can we spend the day as usual, when treasures are strewn along the way? One must become accustomed to the unusual manifestation of life.

407. The Teaching, based on experience, gives to each thinker the joy of application. Hence, let us not demean that which is immeasurably great and near in the flux of our consciousness. Let us not confine in predetermined bounds that which descends as the Breath of the Mother of the World. Let us say how joyful it is to serve the regeneration without fear of the wrong path. Beginning

with the most obvious and the tangible, following the immutable laws, let us apply the best attention to the Teaching of Life.

604. The ancient ones said, "The Mountain of the Mother extends from the earth to the Heavens," indicating thus the unity of all that exists.

620. The Mountain of the Mother of the World does not know its summit. Shall we fear it? Shall we be terrified at its unapproachability? Or shall we rejoice that the Amrita is inexhaustible? Among the concepts of mensurability the Incalculable radiates like light. Shall we be displeased by the coolness of the far-off wind, engendered in Infinity? In the sweltering sterility let us not turn away from a reviving stream.

623. I shall say, translating the hymns of the Mother of the World into life, that you must learn to affirm the origin in the beauty of Cosmos.

640. Beside the radiance of the Mother of the World, the evidence of our existence is like a grain of sand; but the cumulation of the Chalice is like a radiant mountain.

647. The adoption of Our Covenants must be expressed in an undeferrableness of actions. The disciple must not appease himself with a bad result and a good intention. As heavy weights on the scale are light-mindedness, negligence and the demeaning of the Command.

The disciple himself will thrice look into the mirror and say: "I see no mistakes in my actions."

Do not direct thine eye into the plains, but turn to the heights of the Mother of the World, and thus measure limitlessly thine actions.

2. Is it so difficult for the consciousness to propel itself to that source the streams of which are endless? Can the obstacles be so resistive when the Teaching says that it is easy to lift the curtain of the future? Decide to apply this to life, so that the ability to make use of Our advices should not be limited to exclamations or assurances, and let your spirit say, "The wisdom of the Lord is the power of the far-off worlds. The Fire of Infinity and the radiation of the Star of the Mother of the World are sending to us the affirmation of our being!"

7. Eternally moving, eternally striving, eternally aspiring to the heights, eternally manifesting vigilance, affirming Truth, manifesting the radiant thread of the Mother of the World by the armor of infinite beauty, assailing the darkness of ignorance, promising to the abode of humanity the glory of the stars—thus walk, saying, "World, I wish to accept all thy gifts; I wish to fill to the brim the chalice of attainment; I wish, O Lord, to drain the chalice of the wisdom of Thy Covenants!"

9. Why does there exist in the world the custom of worshipping the cosmic powers in the moment of distress? Why only then the attraction toward Infinity? Why just then the recognition of the so-called supernatural forces? I advise that the Name of the Mother of the World be pronounced not as a symbol but as a power-giver. I advise that the Source of Infinity be invoked not as a symbol but as a manifestation of Eternity, as an eternal Generator of beauty and the Creator of the firmament.

10. The cosmic Breath of the Mother of the World is all-pervading. Verily, all is imbued with it. From infin-

itesimal grains of dust to immeasurable magnitudes, life moves and breathes by this Breath. How then not to cognize the power which moves the Universe! How not to ponder upon the essence of Being! Fathom the rhythm of cosmic energy and understand the rhythm of evolution. The essence of evolution is unalterable and is measured by the manifestation of Infinity.

You who fear the end, turn your face to the radiance of the Mother of the World and affirm yourself in the understanding of evolution. There is no limit to the sendings from the Mountains. There is no limit to the warranty of the far-off worlds. There is no limit to the natural treasures of the visible and invisible spheres.

13. How simply people accept the immutability of the rhythm of day and night! Why do we not apply this same conception toward the foundation of our human cycle? Macrocosm and microcosm reflect one and the same manifestation. Why, then, do people try to convince themselves of an eternal night, when they await so simply the coming day? . . .

And where will be the night? Where you seem to perceive its hush the hymns to the Mother of the World begin. Neither day nor night—only Her Radiance!

18. Verily, the beauty of striving toward limitless encompassment will provide a radiant rainbow, and we shall say, "Mother of the World, All-bestowing, All-embracing, we wish to adorn our far-off firmament!"

22. Thou, spirit, striving to the Creator of Cosmos, turn to the Mother of the World. Proclaim what thou seest. Space is revealed as manifesting the utmost creativeness. The immensity of Space and the inalienability of the cosmic forces enrich the kernel of our being. The

levers of evolution are the finest energies which may become the possession of men.

36. The veil of the radiance of the Mother of the World will be the crown of our striving....

Let us look at the one who consciously strives to the veil of the Mother of the World. We shall see that, of all the inexhaustible, numberless consciousnesses, this warrior, aflame with cosmic fires, is borne there where the power of Infinity glows. But here on Earth the warrior carries a brimming chalice. Wondrous is the transposition of our conception thitherward, into our true life!

38. The symbol of the Mother of the World, giving form and purpose to the entire Breath of Cosmos, transforming the kernel into incalculable manifestations, crowns our Earth with beauty.

The Mother of the World is the great creative force in our being.

"Thou hast abided in the cults of the ancients as earth, as sun, as fire, as air, as water.

Thou, the All-bestowing!

Thou, the All-revealing!

Thou who hast made manifest to humanity the great and joyous realization of the Mother!

Thou who hast indicated achievement and who hast veiled thy Image!

Thou who hast manifested to us the Eire of Space!

Thou who hast taken upon thy shoulders the burden of human actions!

We beseech Thee, restore to us our lost smile! Grant us mastery of the sacred Fiery Might!"

47. The spirit, peering into Infinity, will say, "Our

task is only of this urgent hour; our task concerns only reality; but all worlds, formed and unformed, attract us. And the task of the New World is not terrifying, since we endeavor to affirm a new spatial thought."

The Mother of the World lives and constructs. And We proclaim not the utopia envisioned by humanity but a true striving toward endless construction.

49. Cosmic Justice is aware of the design of evolution, and the plan is executed in accordance with the design of one and the same law of the Fire of the Mother of the World.

Let the Fiery Flame illumine mankind!

57. The finding of Materia Lucida on the earthly sphere is possible only in spiritual consciousness. Clumsy hands may not touch the veil of the Mother of the World. A crude consciousness may not formulate the manifestation of cosmic energy. Only the yearning to perceive provides the access to higher matter.

61. The far-off worlds are our manifested path. The far-off worlds are our enlightenment. The far- off worlds are our vistas of the mighty vision of the Mother of the World. The human spirit seeking expansion finds the manifested far-off worlds. Let us say that the unattainable may become attainable and that privation may become wealth. Therefore, let us direct our will to Infinity, in all its beauty.

67. When We assert that the creativeness of Cosmos is diffused in humanity, it means that only individual striving can propel one to that attainment which the Mother of the World and We Arhats proclaim as the higher Sacrament.

Cognition of the fiery energy gives direction to the

spatial principle, but different degrees of tension of the consciousnesses often impede the unification. The triumph of Cosmos is in the harmonization of two Origins.

68. An unbroken path is open to the spirit; it reveals the symbol of the Mother of the World to him who has chosen the symbol of Light. But the erring one who seeks darkness will not touch the Fire of Space.

Attain the understanding of the symbol of the Mother of the World!

79. Humanity has violated the law of cooperation and is expiating this transgression. Each Lord brought back to the planet the balance which had been lost, but the human spirit is so impregnated with the feeling of antagonism that it cannot reach the goal designated by the Lord. Thus, humanity is developing dreadful controversies; and waves will engulf the thinking, which is violated by the denial of Light as the Mother of the World.

96. Life is comprised of an eternal succession of ideas and of manifestations of cosmic energies. How can a spirit who does not project his thought into the realm of ideas adopt the concept of Infinity! When thought will take on the significance of something vital and realizable, it will reveal to man where is joy and where is truth. The quests of thought have led to unification with the Fire of Space. The quests of thought have led to the acceptance of the records of the past. The quests of thought will lead to the realization of higher worlds. The quests of thought will lead to the irradiance of the Mother of the World. Striving will lead to boundless beauty!

115. For an Arhat, annihilation does not exist. Cosmic creation knows no annihilation. The Mother of the World knows no annihilation. Only regeneration will

create that precious chain which extends endlessly. In calling the yielding of the lowest to the highest "transmutation," We wish to affirm the human consciousness in the process of advancement toward Infinity.

117. All the subtlest spiritual manifestations, which affirm the most worthy human actions, We call

Fire. Beauty of achievement lies at the basis of spirit-creativeness. Our Mother of the World has endowed the world with that eternal achievement which is laid into the foundation of the Universe....

The self-sacrificing achievement of the Mother of the World is reflected in spirit-creativeness as the refulgence of Cosmos.

120. An unusual manifestation of psycho-life is in the blending of the Human Atom. It is manifested consciously, and the psycho-dynamic force draws the most subtle threads into the blending. This manifested junction of the separated halves of the Atom is called the Sacred Action of Cosmos. Therefore, Our cosmic mission is sacred, fiery, and urgent. When an Atom approaches the blending and is consciously motivated, the Star of the Mother of the World glows most vividly and the higher worlds are jubilant.

The psycho-united Atoms fill Space with the fire of creation. When the psycho-dynamic force brings together the halves which belong to each other, cosmic justice triumphs and Space is atremble with cosmic jubilation.

156. It is truly told about the power of love for humanity. Can one love a garden and despise its flowers? Can one worship the power of beauty and not show respect for love? I attest that the Power adorning Our

Universe is confirmed as Our Mother of the World—the Feminine Origin! Indeed, one may cite many scientific examples indicative of the creative destiny of woman. Those who deny the evidence of woman's creativeness should reflect that woman gives voluntarily. It does not mean that those who possess the rights are the ones who affirm them. Hence is the woman's path termed one of voluntary giving. Certainly in Cosmos everything is interwoven, but humanity transgresses the laws of the Higher Reason. Truly, the Feminine Origin is most beautiful! Verily, the pinnacle of Be-ness cannot exist without the Feminine Origin. How badly people have mutilated the great cosmic laws! How far people have departed from Truth!

The one who possesses the full Chalice We call a voluntary giver.

170. Let us accept the principle of Be-ness as the affirmation of the Highest Reason, and the Cosmic Magnet will unfold as the manifested might of the Mother of the World. This concept can bring a true understanding of the existence of Our Brotherhood, a true understanding of the far-off worlds, and a true understanding of those principles which ordain man as a creator.

178. Urusvati is right—a wondrous truth is in beauty. Cosmos affirms evolution by this formula. Cosmos directs the world to the mastery of beauty. Yes, verily, the Mother of the World possesses the Magnet of Beauty. And wherever the Spatial Fire has collected the fiery affirmation of its forms, the fire of the spirit manifests itself. When the invisible process is revealed to the fiery spirit, it may then be said that the creative transmutation has been confirmed.

180. When one can manifest the creativeness of the spirit which is directed toward the radiance of the Mother of the World, then truly reflected is the world of highest tensions. And the analogy leads to eternal striving into the spheres manifested by the Cosmic Magnet.

201. It is very difficult to determine the boundaries in Cosmos between the so-called passive and the active. If We say that all forces are active, men will find this declaration a paradox. But a higher consciousness can understand how We perceive all forces of the Origins as active. The differentiation is so bereft of subtlety that it is difficult to convey to people about the principle which dwells in the manifested power of Mulaprakriti. Likewise, the principle of life cannot be asserted without the realization of the Feminine Origin. Like the Cosmos, Mulaprakriti is a universal principle. The Origins cannot be regarded as competitive forces; only unification of the forces creates life. And We, in the higher worlds, manifest a consecrated reverence for the Origin which humanity calls passive. Yes, yes, yes! The higher consciousness knows the Truth and We are ready to proclaim this Truth to humanity; but for this, humanity must ascend the higher step. Yes, yes, yes! When each Lord had to be given to the world by a mother, how may one not revere Thee, Mother of the World! When each Spatial Fire has to be made manifest in a form, how may one not revere Her who gives life! Yes, yes, yes! How then may one not accept as the highest manifestation of the Cosmos the power in the intense symbol of the Mother!

When the Tara was affirmed on Earth, the three rays of the Lords reverberated. These facets of cosmic fires can be seen on the Tara by a sensitive eye. These facets

27

are so powerfully revealed that their radiance melts all discovered obstacles. One may truly say that the Radiant Image will give new understanding.

227. We, Brothers of Humanity, battle arduously for the balance and for the instilling of the Principle of the Mother of the World. When the understanding of creation will be confirmed, it will be possible to evince to humanity the creative power of Fire.

Humanity has so greatly violated the Magnet of Be-ness that the construction of new life must be established. Only thus can be stopped the generation of currents which now so completely engulf humanity. We, Brothers of Humanity, battle for the Cosmic Magnet and for the life principle. The time is complex, but great! In tension, amidst humanity's monstrous noncomprehension of the principle of Be-ness, We give a new Covenant. We summon humanity to that Covenant. In that great Covenant lies the principle of Be-ness. We say to humanity, "Venerate the Origins; venerate the Mother of the World; venerate the awesome Covenant of the Cosmic Magnet! Yes, yes, yes!" Thus speaks Maitreya.

240. The cosmic creativeness responds directly to the delineation of all laws of the Mother of the World.

341. Materia Lucida clothes all aspects of the cosmic energies. The flux of the Fire of Space can envelop for manifestation that region which is subject to the cosmic attraction. The seed, strained toward life, is subject to this great law of attraction. When the power of impulse drives the seed toward creative fire, the striving of consciousness bestows life. The consciousness of the energy is the current of fire. How, then, can priority be given to one energy over another when the fiery tension can

occur only in fusion? He who knows the law of Be-ness can affirm that the acknowledgment of the two Origins is the foundation of Cosmos.

375. Self-action must be understood. In it is comprised the entire synthesis of activity. Verily, selfaction is self-realization. When the spirit can discover its seed and discern the shells that surround it, it can comprehend the beauty of Cosmos.

The husk which gathers about the human spirit clogs the paths to affirmation. Therefore, Our coworkers must understand that a husk is not applicable to Our conditions. One must understand the unworthiness of manifesting the garment of spirit as a husk, when We so greatly revere the radiance of the veil of the Mother of the World.

Hierarchy

4. Our Hierarchy lives and develops by the fiery law. We, Arhats, rejoice at the fire of life and, even more, at the growth of the flame of evolution. Future Arhats, completing their earthly accounts on the planet, are co-workers of Us, the Arhats. When Hierarchy is enriched, there is a cosmic festival. The law is one and eternal. The law is confirmed by Cosmos.

We see the radiance of the worlds. We see the accomplished and endless march. We see the radiance of the Mother of the World! Let us conclude in the joy of the endless march.

8. Maitreya wishes to hasten all. Maitreya wishes that all should be successfully accomplished. Maitreya wishes you joy. Maitreya wishes to grant to humanity the gift of the experiment of Agni Yoga. Maitreya wishes to

transmute life on Earth, in the radiance of the Mother of the World.

9. Ruleress, I pronounce Thee the great Coworker of Cosmic Reason. Ruleress, Thou, beyond all cosmic powers, bearest within Thyself the sacred seed which provides radiant life. Ruleress, affirming all manifestations of the Great Reason, Thou art the Bestower of joy of cosmic creativeness. The Ruleress will adorn the aspiring realm with creative fire. Ruleress of Thought, Thou Who invokest life, to Thee We make manifest the radiance of Our Ray. Mother, venerated of the Lords, We carry in Our Heart the fire of Thy Love. In Thy Heart lives the ordaining Ray. In Thy Heart life is conceived, and We shall affirm the Ray of the Ruleress. Yes, yes, yes!

Thus the Cosmos exists in the greatness of the dual Origin. Yes, yes, yes! Thus the Cosmos crowns the dual Origin. Thus the Mother of the World and the Lords build life. Yes, yes, yes! And in boundless striving the Cosmic Magnet welds its sacred parts. Thus We venerate the Ruleress beyond all spheres.

11. To the Brothers of Humanity is assigned the construction of the life of the planet; and They sustain the Ordinance of the great Mother of the World. The music of the spheres resounds when the current of joy is in motion. The music of the spheres fills the space when the heart is stirred to tremor by the cosmic energy. The Heart of Our Brotherhood safeguards for humanity the path toward the General Good.

13. Each Lord has His keynote. The Epoch of Maitreya proclaims the Woman. The manifestation of Maitreya is linked with the confirmation of the Mother of the

World, in past, present and future. The "Book of Life" is beautiful!

18. Your law is based on human cruelty—Our Law is based upon the Heart of the Mother of the World.

23. To Thee, Mother of the World, the law of Existence is made manifest. To Thee, Ruleress, We Brothers of Humanity pay reverence. Thee, Thee, Thee! Thus the blended heart rules the Universe. Yes, yes, yes!

348. The manifestation of events propels one into the future. Therefore Hierarchy must be understood as the life-belt; thus the sign of the Mother of the World may be understood. We shall shout into the ears of the faint-hearted—Hierarchy!!! The Teaching is given at the imperative hour, but one must have ears of an ass not to hear the thunder.

362. The only natural blending with the Highest is through a naturally kindled fire of the heart. Certainly the boiling of the Chalice that is filled to the brim is unavoidable, but this is the burden of the Mother of the World. Remember the ancient image of an infant lying in a chalice. A multitude of scientific signs are transformed into misty symbols, but it is time to study them.

Heart

106. Why are women often awakened to the Subtle World? Because the work of the heart is much subtler, and thus transcendentalism appears easier for them. Verily, the Era of the Mother of the World is based upon the realization of the heart. It is precisely woman alone who can solve the problem of the two worlds. Thus, one may call woman to the understanding through the heart.

This will also be useful primarily because the quality of the heart is eternal.

203. How, then, shall you proceed? Exactly by clinging firmly to Me and imagining yourself in the midst of the ocean, where only the Scarf of the Mother of the World guards one. In the battle with darkness, unprecedented tenacity is necessary to open all the beautiful possibilities.

Fiery World I

401. One may observe to what great extent humanity has departed from the spiritual principle in the last few years. Many books which should have directed people precisely toward the spiritual life failed, on the contrary, even to attract people's attention. But it cannot continue thus. One must by all methods remind people of the essence of spirit. The existence of numerous sects is of no help, leading people into aimless wandering. The nature of Kali Yuga is characterized by a division of the entire organism into its component parts. But the Blessed Mother arises at dawn, in order to gather these scattered parts of the one Being. The Mother of the World attracts the attention of nations and awaits the Star of the Morning.

429. Mind has been symbolized by the sign of Fire. Fiery thinking is the descent of knowledge of the Fiery World. Such descent marked the great epochs, called the Days of the Mother of the World. Even in the history of Earth, one can trace several such epochs. Will not the future bring such a Day of Light if people will realize the uselessness of evil?

440. The bringing of the Fire is the ancient symbol

of the purification of the spirit. The seed of the spirit itself cannot be defiled, but the ship may become covered with barnacles which hinder its sailing. The Fiery Mother understands when the necessity of purifying the seed approaches. The new sowing may be accomplished only with pure seeds.

One must help when the time comes for the Sower to go out into the field.

663. How may one obtain success? Remember, through joy. Not despair but joy. Do not for an instant believe that We debate the probability or improbability of success. Our only thought is, does your joy suffice to quicken the harvest? We always counsel joy. It is necessary to realize and remember that you have succeeded while rejoicing. Certainly this is not the frisking of a calf on the meadow but the creative joy which dissolves all difficulties. The play of the Mother of the World is in joy. She enfolds the enlightened ones in Her veil of joy. Rejoice amidst flowers; and in the midst of snow— equally redolent—also rejoice!

Fiery World II

5. Let us remember the myth about the "Origin of Mountains." When the planetary Creator toiled over the formation of Earth, He gave attention to fertile plains which could provide people with a quiet agriculture. But the Mother of the World said, "Verily, people will find bread and trade in the plains, but when gold will pollute the plains, whither shall go the pure in spirit to gather strength? Either let them have wings, or let them have mountains, in order to escape from gold." And the Creator answered, "It is too early to give wings to

people, they would carry death and destruction. But let us give them mountains. Even if some be afraid of them, for others they will be salvation." Thus, there are two kinds of people—people of the plains and people of the mountains.

6. Let us recall the myth about the "Origin of Lightning." The Mother of the World said to the Creator, "When Earth will be covered with dark veils of malice, how will the salutary drops of Bliss penetrate?" And the Creator answered, "Torrents of Fire may be gathered which can pierce the thickest layer of darkness." The Mother of the World said, "Verily, the sparks of Eire of Thy Spirit can give salvation, but who will collect and guard them for use when needed?" The Creator replied, "Trees and herbs will preserve My sparks, but when the leaves fall off, then let the deodar and its sisters preserve throughout the year their accumulations of Fire." Thus in various myths there has been reflected the link with the Higher World.

309. Each traveler can fill space with useful ties. Even in antiquity, the dwellers of a community, after a certain length of time, went separate ways for a while. Such an outspreading fluid network has an enormous salutary significance. One must send not only thoughts but also psychic energy over great distances. The ancients called such a fluid network the fabric of the Mother of the World. Therefore, when the Head of the Community proclaimed the approach of the date of departure, the manifested co-workers rejoiced, for this signified that the net of psychic energy was already strong.

424. The Lights of the Mother of the World resemble the pillars of the aurora borealis.

89. The planetary dates correspond with all the supermundane dates. The dark condition of this planet requires all forces for the affirmation of equilibrium. It is easy to think about the future when the spirit knows the bond of the two Worlds, when the spirit can be successful in its strivings toward the Fiery World. There cannot be an intensification which does not reveal to the spirit the amplitude of the manifest future. In the Subtle World events go on which assist manifestations on Earth. Especially tensed are the strata which are close to Earth. Entire armies are being assembled for events. Entire nations are being armed against the forces of destruction. The Supermundane World will not leave the planet helpless. So, too, the Mother of the World and the Hierarchy of Good and the Fiery Viceroys are mobilizing Their camps. Verily, great is the time solving the earthly destiny—the Heavenly Forces saturate the space. Thus let us remember on the path to the Fiery World.

171. With what is the Heart of the Arhat fed? We say— with love. Only this source knows how to saturate the fiery heart. The great Mother of the World knows this source. Each pure heart knows this source. How, then, are the hearts commerged? We say—with love, that powerful source which converts life into a manifestation of beauty, that source which contains all the subtle energies of the heart.

194. Indeed, if humanity would not violate the manifestation of the First Causes, the foundations of Existence would retain that basis which manifests the beauty of life. Cosmic Right brings understanding of the fact that a one-sided administration of the planet is

plunging it into an abyss. Cosmic Right offers to humanity that Principle which can pierce the darkness. Cosmic Right reveals to the planet the unity of Principles which guides the entire Universe. Cosmic Right reveals the Feminine Principle as a manifested power. Cosmic Right reveals the greatness of the Feminine Principle, which manifests self-renunciation, and before which verily the great Arhats bow themselves. Verily, We reverence the great Feminine Principle. Verily, We reverence the giving Principle which bestows the life of Beauty and of the Heart.

Aum

415. The Mother of the World! It would seem that in one sounding of these words would be made clear the meaning of the grandeur of the concept, but life shows otherwise.

Selections from the

LETTERS OF HELENA ROERICH

on

- MOTHER OF THE UNIVERSE
- MOTHER OF THE WORLD
- SCARF OF THE MOTHER OF THE WORLD
- THE GODDESS DUKKAR
- STAR OF THE MOTHER OF THE WORLD
- EPOCH OF THE MOTHER OF THE WORLD
- WOMAN AS MOTHER OF THE WORLD

MOTHER OF THE UNIVERSE

9 January 1935. There is no life, no expression of spirit, without the Mother of the Universe, the Great Matter of All-Being. The placing of spirit and matter into diametrically opposing positions bred in the ignorant consciousness a fanatical conception of matter as something inferior, whereas in reality spirit and matter are one. Spirit without matter is nothing, and matter is but the crystallization of spirit. The manifested Universe, visible and invisible, from the highest to the lowest, reveals to us the infinite aspects of Radiant Matter. Where there is no matter, there is no life. (*Letters Of Helena Roerich.* Vol. I, New York, Agni Yoga Society, 2017, p.342)

18 June 1935. The Mother of the Universe, or of the manifested Cosmos, can be accepted as one of the Figures of the Holy Trinity. Indeed, there is no religion, except later ecclesiastical Christianity, in which the Feminine Element is not included among the Primates of Be-ness. Thus, the Gnostics also considered the Holy Ghost as a Feminine Element. In the most ancient Teachings, the manifested Trinity of Father, Mother, and Son was considered as an emanation of the highest, eternally hidden Cause; and the latter, in turn, as that of the Causeless Cause. (*Ibid.*, p.448)

MOTHER OF THE WORLD

9 January 1935. How beautiful is the Image of the Mother of the World! So much beauty, self-renunciation and tragedy is in this majestic Image! Aspire in your heart to the Highest, and joy and exultation will enter your soul. (*Ibid.*, p.342)

31 May 1935. In the higher worlds the Feminine Principle is greatly revered, for woman is the personification of self-sacrifice and of eternal giving on the path of difficult human evolution. "Woman went by way of achievement," it was said. Let us not forget how the Hierarchy of Light reveres the Mother of the World! (*Ibid.*, p.420)

18 June 1935. The Mother of the World is at the head of the Great Hierarchy of Light of our planet. . . . Behind each symbol stands a High Individuality, and each symbol covers a great reality. Each Great Individuality has its deputies, or personifiers, who are nearest to its Ray, and sometimes one of these Great Individualities personally incarnates—hence the concept of the Avatar, (*Ibid.*, p.448)

SCARF OF THE MOTHER OF THE WORLD

8 August 1934. You ask about "Khatak of the Mother of the World." "Khatak" is the sacred silk scarf which Mongolians and Tibetans present to all spiritual representatives and all especially revered persons, as a sign of respect. In Buddhist shrines all sacred Images are covered by, or wrapped in, these silk scarves, the length of which varies from one to five yards, and the width from a quarter of a yard to one yard. Their colors are white and yellow in Tibet, and blue and yellow in Mongolia. Sometimes holy Images and happy signs are woven into them. The khatak is a symbol of protection and help. On the sacred paintings of Tibet and Mongolia, the so- called tankas, or banners, one can often see depicted a saint from the Subtle World lowering a khatak to a sinner in the lower spheres, and the latter climbing up the khatak. (*Ibid.*, p.245)

THE GODDESS DUKKAR

17 December 1929. The great time predicted long ago has come. Do you not feel it in all the tension of cosmic and human explosions? All the crust of the earth is aquiver, and a great change is approaching. This time it is not the comparatively harmless tail of a comet but our own emanations which, by their discord with the approaching higher fiery energies, may evoke—or rather will evoke—an unexpected change. It is good during such perturbations to be on the solid indicated rock, under the Umbrella of Dukkar. Our tasks will all have room under this cover. (*Ibid.*, p.26)

24 June 1935. "Dukkar," the many-eyed and many-armed, is a Tibetan Divinity of the Feminine Element. She is an equivalent of the Hindu Kali and Lakshmi, the symbol of the Mother of the World. Usually, on Tibetan tankas, She is represented under an umbrella, which symbolizes the gathered drops of Highest Bliss. (*Ibid.*, p.457)

STAR OF THE MOTHER OF THE WORLD

11 January 1935. The Star of the Mother of the World is the planet Venus. In 1924 this planet for a short time came unusually near to the Earth. Its rays were poured on Earth, and this created many new powerful and sacred combinations which will yield great results. Many feminine movements were kindled by these powerful rays. (*Ibid.*, p.345)

EPOCH OF THE MOTHER OF THE WORLD

1933. It would be very desirable if the members of the Woman's Society could start their work with the tasks of self-perfection and self-education, and would try, with united efforts, to apply them in life. In the coming era of the Mother of the World, great numbers of cultured women are needed—women educated in various branches of knowledge, arts, crafts, etc. Every woman should be also a trained nurse, or at least should know elementary hygiene and medicine. In addition, would it not be wonderful if they could learn also spiritual healing? (*Ibid.*, p.142)

10 October 1934. The New Epoch requires spiritual cognition. The New Epoch must manifest due respect to the Mother of the World, to the Feminine Element. "The bird of the spirit of Humanity cannot fly with only one wing"—these are the words of Vivekananda, who meant to affirm the great significance of the Feminine Principle. Man does not willingly give full rights to woman. However, this opposition but intensifies the forces; and woman, fighting for her cosmic rights, will acquire the knowledge of her power. (*Ibid.*, p.300)

8 March 1933. The equilibrium of the elements is a foundation of Life, and the violation of this law leads to destruction. And now the Great Teachers will affirm the rights of woman. Therefore, the coming epoch will be not only an epoch of great cooperation, it will also be the epoch of Woman. Woman will have to be armed with courage, and, first of all, she will have to restrain her heart from unwise giving, for there must be the Golden Balance in everything. Woman must affirm herself, and that is why the Sword of Spirit is given precisely into the hands of woman. In the East this epoch is noted as the epoch of Maitreya, the epoch of Great Compassion, and the epoch of the Mother of the World, (*Ibid.*, p.376)

WOMAN AS MOTHER OF THE WORLD

1 March 1929. Could the terrors and crimes of today be possible if both Origins had been balanced? In the hands of woman lies the salvation of humanity and of our planet. Woman must realize her significance, the great mission of the Mother of the World; she should be prepared to take responsibility for the destiny of humanity. Mother, the life- giver, has every right to direct the destiny of her children. The voice of woman, the mother, should be heard amongst the leaders of humanity. The mother suggests the first conscious thoughts to her child. She gives direction and quality to all his aspirations and abilities. But the mother who possesses no thought of culture can suggest only the lower expressions of human nature. . . .

Western woman is awake and realizes her powers. Her cultural contributions are already evident. However, the majority of Western women—as with all beginners—start with imitation; whereas, it is in original self-expression that real beauty and harmony are found. Would we like to see man losing the beauty of manhood? The same is true about a man who has a sense of beauty. He certainly does not wish to see a woman imitating his habits and competing with his vices. Imitation always starts with the easiest. But we hope that this first step will soon be outlived and that woman will deepen her knowledge of Mother-Nature and will find true, original ways of self-expression. . . .

The mother, the life-giver, the life-protector—let her become also the Mother, the Leader, the *All*-Giver, the *All*-Receiver. (*Ibid.*, p.13-16)

7 October 1930. Now, let woman—the Mother of the World—say, "Let there be Light," and let her affirm her fiery achievements. What will this Light be like, and which of her achievements will be the great fiery ones? The banner of spirit will be raised, and upon it will be inscribed "Love, Knowledge and Beauty." Yes, only the heart of the woman, the mother, may gather under this Banner the children of the whole world, without distinctions of sex, race, nationality and religion....

Let us, therefore, without delay raise the great Banner of the New Era—the Era of the Mother of the World. Let every woman enlarge the boundaries of her hearth to encompass the hearths of the whole world. These countless fires will strengthen and embellish her own hearth....

Humanity should realize the majestic cosmic law of equivalency, the law of the dual Origin, as the foundation of existence. The predominance of one Origin over the other has created a lack of balance and destruction, which may now be observed in all of life. But let not the woman who has realized this law, and who strives toward equilibrium, let her not lose the beauty of the feminine image; let her not lose tenderness of heart, subtlety of feelings, the self-sacrifice and the courage of patience.

Woman, the bearer of sacred knowledge, can become a calling power, kindling with fiery words the souls that are ready. It is necessary to give to every woman according to her consciousness and without impeding her natural and individual growth. It is necessary, with careful touches, to broaden the mind on the foundation of the Teaching of Life. Let every soul develop in a natural way, bringing out the best she can according to the level of her consciousness. Beauty is in variety, but all should have one general foundation—the foundation of striving toward the General Good. The broadest cooperation is inscribed on the Banner of the Mother of the World. Therefore, let us display the utmost tolerance.

Sisters of the Golden Mountain, a dangerous but beautiful time is ahead of us—a time of great achievements. I send you the call of my heart. Let us arm ourselves with flaming striving and with courage, and over all obstacles we shall carry the Banner of the Mother of the World—the Banner of Love, Self-sacrifice and Beauty—so that in the hour of victory we shall plant it on the Summits of the World. (*Ibid.*, p.44-45)

AGNI YOGA SERIES

Leaves of Morya's Garden I (The Call) 1924

Leaves of Morya's Garden II (Illumination) 1925

New Era Community 1926

Signs of Agni Yoga

Agni Yoga 1929

Infinity I 1930

Infinity II 1930

Hierarchy 1931

Heart 1932

Fiery World I 1933

Fiery World II 1934

Fiery World III 1935

Aum 1936

Brotherhood 1937

Supermundane (in 3 volumes) 1938

Letters of Helena Roerich, Vol. I 1929-1935

Letters of Helena Roerich, Vol. II 1935-1939

AGNI YOGA SOCIETY
www.agniyoga.org

www.ingramcontent.com/pod-product-compliance
Lightning Source LLC
Chambersburg PA
CBHW072157020426
42334CB00018B/2044